EFFECTS AND TREATMENT OF STROKE

WHAT YOU MUST DO TO PREVENT STROKE

John B. Mills

TABLE OF CONTENTS

Chapter 1

STROKE EFFECTS AND TREATMENT

A stroke happens when a blood artery obstruction or hemorrhage stops or lowers the delivery of blood to the brain. When this occurs, the brain receives insufficient oxygen and nutrients, and brain cells begin to die.

A stroke is a kind of cerebrovascular illness. This indicates that it affects the blood arteries that provide oxygen to the brain. Damage to the brain may begin if it does not get enough oxygen.There is a medical emergency here. While many strokes are curable, some might result in disability or death.

A stroke occurs when the blood flow to a portion of the brain is interrupted. Brain cells may be harmed or die in the absence of blood. Stroke may have both short- and long-term consequences, depending on which area of the brain is injured and how fast it is treated. Stroke survivors may have a variety of problems, including challenges with movement and communication, as well as changes in how they think and feel.

Access to therapy as soon as possible saves lives and promotes recovery. If you see any of the symptoms of a stroke, contact an ambulance right once.

Stroke is a condition in which the blood flow to the brain is interrupted, resulting in oxygen deprivation, brain damage, and functional loss. A clot in an artery providing blood to the brain is the most common cause. It may also be caused by hemorrhage, which occurs when a blood artery bursts and causes blood to bleed into the brain.

A stroke may result in lasting damage, such as partial paralysis and impaired speech, understanding, and memory. The kind and degree of impairment are impacted by the portion of the brain injured and the amount of time the blood supply has been cut off.

The prevalence of stroke has already reached pandemic proportions.

One in every four persons over the age of 25 will suffer a stroke throughout their lives. This year, 12.2 million individuals will suffer their first stroke, and 6.5 million will die as a consequence. Over 110 million individuals worldwide have had a stroke.

Stroke incidence rises dramatically with age, yet over 60% of strokes occur in adults under the age of 70, and 16% occur in people under the age of 50.

High blood pressure as a consequence of atherosclerosis is a major clinical risk factor for stroke. Tobacco usage, physical inactivity, an unhealthy diet, dangerous alcohol use, atrial fibrillation, elevated blood cholesterol levels, obesity, hereditary tendency, stress, and depression are all risk factors.

SYMPTOMS OF A STROKE

Knowing the symptoms of a stroke and getting urgent emergency medical treatment may save lives and improve survivors' outcomes. People who have had a stroke may have

- Facial drooping
- Arm weakness on one side
- Speech issues - slurring or not making sense
- Changes in eyesight
- Loss of balance/dizziness.

Chapter 2

EFFECTS OF STROKE

The repercussions of a stroke vary depending on the kind, severity, location, and frequency of strokes. The brain is very complicated. Each part of the brain is in charge of a certain function or aptitude.

When a stroke damages a section of the brain, a component of the body's regular function may be lost. This might lead to a handicap.

The brain is split into three sections:

1. Cerebrum (right and left halves or hemispheres) (right and left sides or hemispheres)

2. Cerebellum (top and front of the brain) (top and front of brain)

3. Brainstem (base of the brain) (base of the brain)

The symptoms of a stroke might vary greatly depending on which of these areas of the brain is affected.

Cerebrum, cerebellum, and brainstem location:

1. The cerebrum is the section of the brain located at the top and front of the skull. It is in charge of movement and sensation, as well as speaking, thinking, reasoning, memory, vision, and emotions. The cerebrum is split into right and left halves, sometimes known as hemispheres.

Any or all of the following functions may be compromised depending on the location and side of the cerebrum affected by the stroke:

- Sensation and movement
- Language and Speech
- Consuming and swallowing
- Vision
- Cognitive capacity (thinking, reasoning, judgment, and remembering)

- Perception and orientation to the environment
- Self-care skills
- Control of the bowel and bladder
- Controlling one's emotions
- Sexual prowess

Aside from these broad impacts, specific abnormalities may develop when a specific section of the cerebrum is destroyed.

Cerebral effects of a right hemisphere stroke:

1. A right hemisphere stroke may have the following consequences:
    - Sensory impairment with left-sided weakness or paralysis Denial of paralysis or disability, as well as a lack of understanding of the issues caused by the stroke (this is called "left neglect"),
    - Visual issues, such as the inability to view the left visual field of each eye,
    - Depth perception or orientation issues, such as up or down and front or back,

- Inability to locate or identify bodily components,
- Inability to read maps and locate goods such as clothes or toiletries
- Memory issues,
- Changes in behavior such as a lack of care for circumstances, impulsivity, inappropriateness, and sadness.

Cerebral effects of a left hemisphere stroke:

A left hemisphere stroke may have the following consequences:

- Sensory impairment and right-sided weakness or Speech and language comprehension issues (aphasia)
- Visual issues, such as an inability to view the right visual field of each eye
- Impaired capacity to perform arithmetic, organize, reason, and analyze information
- Depression, cautiousness, and reluctance are examples of behavioral alterations.

- Inability to read, write, or learn new information Memory issues

2. The cerebellum is placed near the rear of the skull, under and behind the cerebrum. Through the spinal cord, it gets sensory information from the body. It aids in the synchronization of muscular activity and control, as well as delicate movement, coordination, and balance.

Although cerebellar strokes are less frequent, the consequences may be severe. Cerebellar strokes have four frequent consequences:

- Inability to walk as well as coordination and balance issues (ataxia)
- Dizziness
- Headache
- Vomiting and nausea

3. The brainstem is placed at the brain's base, just above the spinal cord. The brainstem controls many of the body's key "life-support" activities, such as heartbeat, blood pressure, and breathing. It also aids in the regulation of the key

nerves responsible for eye movement, hearing, speaking, chewing, and swallowing. Some of the most prevalent side effects of a brainstem stroke include:

- Breathing and cardiovascular functions
- Body temperature regulation
- Coordination and balance
- Paralysis or weakness
- Chewing, swallowing, and communicating
- Vision

Unfortunately, brainstem strokes may result in death.

Chapter 3

RISK FACTORS AND CAUSES OF STROKE

A stroke, also known as a brain attack, occurs when blood flow to the brain is interrupted. It is a life-threatening circumstance.

To function properly, the brain requires a steady supply of oxygen and nutrients. Even a little interruption in blood flow might create complications. After just a few minutes without blood or oxygen, brain cells begin to die.

Brain function is lost when brain cells die. You may be unable to do tasks that are controlled by that region of your brain. A stroke, for example, may impair your ability to:
Move, Speak, eat, reflect, and remember,
Maintain control over your bowel and bladder.
Maintain emotional control.
Other critical physiological processes within your control.
A stroke may strike anybody at any moment.

CAUSES OF STROKE

A stroke occurs when blood flow to the brain is interrupted or halted.

Stroke has two basic causes: ischemic and hemorrhagic.

1. Stroke caused by ischemia:

   This kind of stroke is the most prevalent. It occurs when a major blood artery in the brain becomes clogged. A blood clot might obstruct it. It might also be clogged by an accumulation of fatty deposits and cholesterol. This accumulation is known as plaque.

2. Stroke caused by hemorrhage: This happens when a blood artery in your brain breaks, causing blood to leak into adjacent tissues. Pressure builds up in adjacent brain tissue during a

hemorrhagic stroke. This creates further harm and discomfort.

A stroke may happen to anybody at any age. However, if you have specific risk factors, your chances of having a stroke rise. Some stroke risk factors can be adjusted or controlled, while others cannot.

Risk factors for stroke that may be altered, treated, or controlled medically include:

1. When their blood pressure is high. Blood vessels (arteries) that feed blood to the brain may be damaged by blood pressure of 140/90 or greater.
2. Cardiovascular disease: Heart disease is the second leading cause of stroke and the leading cause of mortality among stroke survivors. Many of the risk factors for heart disease and stroke are the same.
3. Diabetes. People with diabetes are more likely to have a stroke than those who do not have diabetes.

4. Smoking. Smoking almost doubles your chance of having an ischemic stroke.
5. Pills for birth control (oral contraceptives)

The Origins of TIAs (transient ischemic attacks). Mini-strokes are another term for TIAs. They exhibit the same symptoms as stroke, although the symptoms are transient. If you've had one or more TIAs, you're almost ten times more likely to have a stroke than someone your age and gender who hasn't had a TIA

Red blood cell count is elevated. A considerable increase in the number of red blood cells thickens the blood and increases the likelihood of clotting. This increases the likelihood of having a stroke.

High blood cholesterol and lipid levels: High cholesterol levels may lead to artery thickening or hardening (atherosclerosis) caused by plaque accumulation.

Plaque is a buildup of fatty acids, cholesterol, and calcium. Plaque accumulation on the interior of the arterial walls may reduce blood flow to the brain. A stroke happens when the brain's blood supply is cut off.

- Lack of physical activity
- Obesity
- Excessive alcohol consumption. More than two alcoholic beverages each day elevates blood pressure, drinking may result in a stroke.
- Illegal drugs. IV (intravenous) drug misuse increases the risk of stroke due to blood clots (cerebral embolisms). Cocaine and other narcotics have been linked to strokes, heart attacks, and a variety of other cardiovascular issues.
- A typical cardiac beat. Some forms of heart disease might increase your chances of having a stroke. The most potent and modifiable cardiac risk factor for stroke is an abnormal heartbeat (atrial fibrillation).
- Heart structural abnormalities: Long-term (chronic) heart damage may be caused by damaged heart valves

(valvular heart disease). This may increase your risk of stroke over time.

Unchangeable stroke risk factors include:

1. Getting older: After the age of 55, your chances of suffering a stroke are more than double.
2. Race: African Americans are far more likely than whites to die or be disabled as a result of a stroke. This is due in part to the African-American population's higher prevalence of hypertension.
3. Gender: A stroke occurs more often in males, although stroke kills more women than men.
4. Previous stroke history: You are more likely to suffer a second stroke if you have previously had one.
5. Genetics or heredity: People who have a family history of stroke are more likely to get one.

Other risk factors are:

- Where you reside. Strokes are more prevalent in the southern United States than in other regions. This might be due to variances in lifestyle, race, smoking habits, and food.
- Climate, season, and temperature: Stroke fatalities are more common in severe temperatures.
- Factors of social and economic importance: Strokes seem to be more prevalent among low-income persons, according to some studies.

Chapter 4

SIGNS AND SYMPTOMS OF A STROKE

A stroke is a medical emergency. It is critical to recognize the symptoms of a stroke and get medical attention as soon as possible. When treatment is started as soon as possible, it is most effective.

Stroke symptoms might appear unexpectedly. The symptoms of each individual may differ. Symptoms could include:

1. Weakness or numbness of the face, arm, or leg, often on one side of the body.
2. Difficulties speaking or comprehending.
3. Eyesight issues, such as dimness or loss of vision in one or both eyes
4. Dizziness or balance or coordination issues
5. Movement or walking difficulties
6. Seizures or fainting (loss of consciousness)
7. Severe headaches with no known reason, particularly if they occur unexpectedly.

8. Sudden nausea, or vomiting not caused by viral illness
9. Fainting, disorientation, convulsions, or coma.
10. A brief loss or alteration of consciousness.

TIA, often known as a mini-stroke

Many of the symptoms of a TIA are similar to those of a stroke. However, TIA symptoms are temporary. They might last as little as a few minutes or as long as 24 hours. If you suspect someone is experiencing a TIA, call 911 immediately. It might be a clue that a stroke is on its way. However, not all TIAs result in a stroke.

Seek assistance FAST
FAST is a simple approach to memorizing the symptoms of a stroke. When you observe these indicators. FAST is an abbreviation for:

F - Drooping of the brow. One side of the face droops or is numb. When the individual grins, the smile is uneven.

A - Weakness in the arm. One of your arms is weak or numb. When a person elevates both arms simultaneously, one arm may slide downward.

S - Difficulty speaking. Slurred speech or difficulty speaking may be seen. When questioned, the individual cannot accurately repeat a simple statement.

T - It's time to dial 911. If you see any of these signs, contact 911 immediately. Even if the symptom goes away, call. Keep track of when the symptoms initially arose.

HOW IS A STROKE IDENTIFIED?

Your healthcare professional will conduct a thorough health history and physical assessment. You will need stroke testing such as brain imaging and assessing blood flow in the brain. Among the possible tests are:

1. CT scan of the brain: An X-ray imaging technique that produces crisp, detailed

pictures of the brain. A brain CT scan may detect bleeding in the brain or brain cell damage caused by a stroke. It is used to detect anomalies and aid in determining the site or kind of stroke.

2. MRI. This test creates comprehensive pictures of organs and structures in the body by combining huge magnets, radiofrequency, and a computer. An MRI employs magnetic fields to detect minute changes in brain tissue that aid in the detection and diagnosis of stroke.
3. CTA (computed tomographic angiography) (computed tomographic angiography). The blood vessels as seen on an X-ray. A CT angiography is a procedure that employs CT technology to create pictures of blood arteries.
4. MRA (magnetic resonance angiography) (magnetic resonance angiography). This examination uses MRI technology to assess blood flow via the arteries.
5. Doppler ultrasound (carotid ultrasound). A test that uses sound waves to provide images of the inside of your carotid arteries. This test may determine whether

or not plaque has constricted or obstructed your carotid arteries.

The following cardiac tests may also be done to assist in the diagnosis of heart issues that may have resulted in a stroke:

- Electrocardiogram (ECG). This test measures the electrical activity of your heart. It reveals any abnormal cardiac rhythms that may have contributed to a stroke.

- Echocardiography. This test creates an image of your heart using sound waves. This examination determines the size and shape of your heart. It may determine whether or not the heart valves are functioning appropriately. It may also detect blood clots inside your heart.

WHAT IS THE TREATMENT FOR A STROKE

Your healthcare practitioner will develop a treatment plan for you based on the following factors:

Your age, general health, and medical history

The sort of stroke you experienced

How bad was your stroke

Where in your brain did the stroke occur?

What exactly triggered your stroke

How well do you tolerate certain medications, treatments, or therapies

Once a stroke has happened, there is no cure. However, cutting-edge medicinal and surgical therapies are available. These may help lower your chances of having another stroke.

When treatment is started as soon as possible, it is most effective. Following a stroke, emergency care may include:

1. Anti-clotting medications (thrombolytics or fibrinolytics). These drugs dissolve blood clots, which cause an ischemic stroke. They may aid in the reduction of brain cell damage induced by a stroke. They must be administered within 3 hours following a stroke to be most helpful.
2. Treatment and medications to minimize or manage brain swelling. Special IV (intravenous) fluids are often utilized to minimize or regulate brain edema. They are very useful after a hemorrhagic stroke.
3. Neuroprotective drugs These medications assist to protect the brain from injury and oxygen deficiency (ischemia).
4. Life-saving methods These therapies include breathing assistance from a machine (a ventilator), IV fluids, adequate nutrition, and blood pressure management.

5. Craniotomy: This is a form of brain surgery used to remove blood clots, alleviate pressure, or heal brain hemorrhage.

What are the risks of having a stroke?

The size and location of the stroke influence stroke recovery and the particular ability impacted.

A little stroke might result in complications such as an arm or leg paralysis.

Larger strokes may cause sections of your body to become immobile (paralyzed). Larger strokes might result in speech loss or even death.

What can I do to avoid having a stroke?

Understand your stroke risk. Many risk factors for stroke may be altered, managed, or medically adjusted. The following are some things you can take to manage your risk factors.

1. Changes in lifestyle: A healthy lifestyle may help lower your chance of having a stroke. This contains the following items:
2. If you smoke, you should stop.
3. Make nutritious food choices. Consume the recommended portions of fruits, vegetables, and whole grains. Reduce your consumption of saturated fat, trans fat, cholesterol, salt (sodium), and added sweets.
4. Maintain a healthy weight.
5. Engage in some physical activity.
6. Limit your alcohol consumption.
7. Medicines: Take your medications exactly as prescribed by your doctor. The following medications may aid in stroke prevention:
8. Blood-thinning medications (anticoagulants) aid in the prevention of blood clot formation. Regular blood tests may be required if you use a blood thinner.
9. Many stroke patients are given antiplatelet medications, such as aspirin. They reduce the likelihood of blood clot

formation. Aspirin is accessible without a prescription.

10. Blood pressure medications aid in the reduction of high blood pressure. You may need to take more than one blood pressure medication.
11. Cholesterol-reducing medications make plaque less likely to form in your arterial walls, decreasing your risk of stroke.
12. Certain heart disorders that raise your risk of stroke may be treated with cardiac medications.
13. Diabetes medications regulate blood sugar levels. This may help to avoid complications that might lead to a stroke.
14. Surgery: Several forms of surgery may be performed to treat or prevent a stroke. These are some examples:
15. Endarterectomy of the aorta: Carotid endarterectomy is a procedure used to remove plaque and clots from the carotid arteries in the neck. These arteries carry blood from the heart to the brain. Endarterectomy may aid in the prevention of a stroke.

16. Carotid stenting: A big metal coil (stent) is inserted into the carotid artery in the same way as a stent is inserted into the coronary artery.
17. Aneurysm and AVM repair surgery (arteriovenous malformations): An aneurysm is a weakened, inflated region on the wall of an artery. It has the potential to burst (rupture) and cause bleeding in the brain. An AVM is a twisted network of arteries and veins. It obstructs blood circulation and puts you in danger of bleeding.
18. Closure of a patent foramen ovale (PFO). The foramen ovale is a hole in the wall between the two upper chambers of the heart. This gap normally resolves shortly after delivery. Clots and air bubbles might enter the cerebral circulation if the flap does not shut. This may result in a stroke or TIA (transient ischemic attack). Experts are still divided on whether the PFO should be shuttered.

Suffering from a stroke?

The location of the stroke in your brain determines how it affects you. It also relies on the extent of your brain injury. Many stroke victims have paralysis of one of their arms. Other issues that might arise include:

- Thinking
- Speaking
- Swallowing
- Simple arithmetic tasks such as adding, subtracting, and balancing a checkbook
- Dressing
- Showering
- Using the restroom

Some individuals may need long-term physical therapy. They may be unable to live in their house without assistance.

Following a stroke, support services are provided to assist with physical and emotional requirements.

When should I contact my physician?

- Strokes may occur again. Call your doctor if you experience symptoms that resemble a stroke, even if they are brief.

- If you sustain recurrent brain tissue injury, you may develop life-long (permanent) problems.

Key points of the stroke

A stroke occurs when blood flow to the brain is interrupted. It is a life-threatening circumstance.

A restricted blood artery, hemorrhage, or a clot that inhibits blood flow may all cause it.

Symptoms might appear unexpectedly. Call 911 immediately if you suspect someone is having a stroke.

If you get emergency care straight away, you have a greater chance of recovering from a stroke.

The way a stroke affects you is determined by where the stroke happens in your brain and the extent to which your brain is injured.

Chapter 5

WHAT YOU CAN DO TO PREVENT STROKE

You may help avoid stroke by making healthy choices and managing any existing health concerns.

1. Living a healthy lifestyle: Many strokes might be avoided by adopting a healthy lifestyle and working with your healthcare team to treat health issues that increase your chance of having a stroke. Making good lifestyle choices may help avoid stroke.

2. Take Initiative and Be Inspired: Find advice and tools to help you make the best health decisions for you. "Begin Small. "Live Largely." external symbol This advertisement urges seniors, 55 and older to get back on track by taking little measures, such as making medical

appointments, getting active, and eating healthy, so they may live large again.

3. "Beat it to the Beat."external symbol: This campaign aims to inspire Black adults to live heart-healthy lives on their terms, and to discover what works best for them individually and consistently as they live to their rhythm.
4. Choose nutritious meals and beverages: Choosing healthy meals and snacks selections may aid in stroke prevention. Consume lots of fresh fruits and vegetables.
5. Eating meals rich in fiber and low in saturated fat, trans fat, and cholesterol may help avoid high cholesterol. Limiting your salt (sodium) intake may also help reduce your blood pressure. High blood pressure and high cholesterol both raise your chances of having a stroke.
6. Maintain a healthy weight: Obesity and being overweight raise your risk of stroke. Doctors often analyze your body mass index to see if your weight is within a healthy level (BMI). If you know your weight and height, you may use the

CDC's Assessing Your Weight website to determine your BMI. Doctors may occasionally use waist and hip measurements to determine extra body fat.

7. Engage in frequently physical exercise: Physical exercise may help you maintain a healthy weight while also lowering your cholesterol and blood pressure. The surgeon general advises 2 hours and 30 minutes of moderate-intensity aerobic physical exercise per week for adults, such as a brisk stroll. Every day, children and teenagers should engage in one hour of physical exercise.
8. Do not smoke: Cigarette smoking significantly raises your risk of getting a stroke. Don't start smoking if you don't already. If you smoke, stopping will reduce your chance of having a stroke. Your doctor may advise you on how to stop smoking.
9. Consume alcohol in moderation: Drinking too much alcohol might cause your blood pressure to rise. Men should limit themselves to two drinks each day,

while women should limit themselves to one.

10. Maintain control of your medical circumstances: Consult your doctor about ways to reduce your chance of a stroke.
11. You can reduce your risk of stroke if you have heart disease, high cholesterol, high blood pressure, or diabetes.
12. Examine your cholesterol levels: Your cholesterol levels should be checked by your doctor at least once every five years. Discuss this easy blood test with your medical staff. If you have high cholesterol, medication and lifestyle modifications may help reduce your stroke risk.
13. Maintain blood pressure control: Because high blood pressure normally has no symptoms, get it tested regularly. Consult your doctor about how often you should check your levels. You may have your blood pressure checked at home, at the doctor's office, or the drugstore. If you have high blood pressure, your doctor may give medication, suggest lifestyle

modifications, or advise you to eat foods with less sodium (salt).

14. Diabetes management: If your doctor suspects you have diabetes, he or she may advise you to be tested. Check your blood sugar levels regularly if you have diabetes.
15. Discuss treatment choices with your medical team. Your doctor may advise you to make specific lifestyle adjustments, such as increasing your physical activity or eating healthier foods. These activities can help you maintain appropriate blood sugar management and minimize your risk of stroke.
16. Treat cardiovascular disease: Your healthcare provider may propose medical therapy or surgery if you have certain cardiac issues, such as coronary artery disease or atrial fibrillation (irregular heartbeat). Taking care of cardiac issues may aid in stroke prevention.
17. Take your medication as directed: If you are taking medication to treat heart disease, high cholesterol, high blood pressure, or diabetes, carefully follow

your doctor's recommendations. If you don't understand anything, always ask questions. Never discontinue your medication without first consulting your doctor or pharmacist.

18. Collaborate with your medical team: You and your medical team can collaborate to prevent or cure the medical issues that contribute to stroke. Bring a list of questions to your sessions and discuss your treatment plan frequently. Find the perfect doctor for your external symbol from the "Live to the Beat" campaign

If you've previously had a stroke or TIA, your healthcare team will collaborate with you to avoid future strokes. Your treatment strategy will involve medication or surgery as well as lifestyle modifications to reduce your chance of having another stroke. Take your medication exactly as advised and follow your doctor's instructions.

www.ingramcontent.com/pod-product-compliance
Lightning Source LLC
LaVergne TN
LVHW020532160826
845677LV00015B/4023